Mammograms Mastectomies and A Spiritual Makeover

Jill Nogales

Jebaire Publishing, LLC
Snellville, GA

ISBN-10: 0-9786796-1-x
ISBN-13: 978-0-9786796-1-3
Library of Congress Control Number: 2011903052

Interior Editor: Fran Lowe
Supervising Editor: Shannon Clark
Cover Design: Jebaire Publishing
Back Cover Photo by Marilyn Markus

Visit Jill Nogales' website at:
www.anewshadeofpink.wordpress.com

Visit Jebaire's website at:
www.jebairepublishing.com

Jebaire Publishing is an independent, non-denominational Christian book publisher. We are a free press and report to no outside groups. Our mission is to provide relevant Christian resources that both inspire and encourage our readers to pursue a meaningful relationship with Jesus Christ.

NOTE: The views expressed in this book are of a personal nature. Readers should consult the appropriate healthcare professional for any matter related to their health and well being.

Dedication

To all the women whose lives have been turned upside down by cancer. May God lavish upon you His extraordinary gifts.

Table of Contents

Introduction

Are You Crazy, Mom?

Abreast cancer diagnosis does not exactly make a woman want to turn cartwheels, yet some good can come from this horrible ordeal. Really. I discovered it for myself when my first-ever routine mammogram indicated advanced, invasive cancer. The good thing is that when you have cancer, God Himself takes the opportunity to lavish you with His extraordinary gifts-- gifts such as grace, courage, peace, and joy.

When I first told my family that I intended to write a book about the good that can come from breast cancer, my nine-year-old son Connor said, "Are you crazy, Mom? There is *nothing* good about cancer!"

Of course, he is absolutely right; there is nothing good about breast cancer. But you *can* make a choice about which attitude to adopt. You can either choose defeat, resentment, or self-pity, or you can choose to look on the bright side of a really awful situation. I like to think of it as a spiritual makeover. When you get cancer, your physical well-being demands all the attention. In the battle to save your body, it's often easy to neglect the damage cancer can do to your spirit.

The amazing thing about having your life turned upside down by cancer is that God stays so wonderfully close. He sees your tears, feels your pain, and knows your heartache. He has already antici- pated your every need before you even take the first step of your cancer journey.

Let me share God's extravagant gifts with you and encourage you to discover them for yourself. Breast cancer is not a journey any one of us would have chosen; however, as long as we're going that way, let's take a break from the bad stuff to discover the good gifts God has prepared for us. Let's give ourselves a spiritual makeover.

"Every good and perfect gift is from above, coming down from the Father of the heavenly lights." (James 1:17)

"And we know that in all things God works for the good of those who love him." (Rom. 8:28a)

1

GRACE

A Love Letter from God

Few words are as life-changing as "You have cancer." When I first heard those words, I became horribly aware that life as I knew it would never, ever be the same.

People, with kind intentions no doubt, would come up to me, pat my hand, and say, "I know what you're going through. I had a lump," or "I had a suspicious mammogram too." Each time I heard words like these, I had to fight an incredibly strong urge to whack them in the nose…hard, because there is a gargantuan difference between finding out that the lump was benign or the mammogram was okay after all— and finding out you have cancer.

Our minds are not equipped to handle this kind of news with ease. While my brain struggled to process this whole cancer thing, life actually continued to go on. How could my life get dumped upside down, and yet life around me moved forward, just like normal? My children still needed to be cared for and put to bed. Groceries had to be purchased and meals cooked. Dishes and laundry got dirty and required washing. How could this be?

I would be pushing a grocery cart when all of a sudden it would come to my mind: *I have cancer.* While driving down the road, running errands like I have done for years, I would suddenly remember that *I have cancer.* Every time I remembered, I experienced the shock of the initial diagnosis all over again. Eventually I found it easier to think about the cancer all the time, because if I did forget about it for a little while, the reality of my diagnosis would come back and hit me like a train.

As the primary shock wore off, one question began to swirl in my mind. *What in the world could I have done to have caused this?* I have always tried my best to avoid close contact with pesticides, toxic materials, and electromagnetic fields, as well as any other noxious substances of a suspicious nature. All my life, thanks to my mom, I have been a healthy eater. In fact, I eat bananas and wheat bread every day, and I don't even *like* bananas or wheat bread. I exercise regularly, even on the days when I don't feel like it. I have no family history of cancer. So how could I have possibly ended up with this disease?

The one answer that came to mind was that I must be a really awful person, because only a really awful person deserves to have breast cancer. Of course, *now* I know that's not true, but at the time, it made complete sense to me. My brain started operating like a computer stuck in a loop. Over and over again, a voice in my head said, "You deserve to have breast cancer."

One of the ladies I knew from church cried when she first heard about my cancer. "This is big, Jill," she said. "We have to tell everyone. You are going to need lots of support."

"No," I whispered. "I don't want anyone to know."

"But, Jill," she insisted, "everyone is going to know you have cancer when your hair falls out!"

It's funny what comes surging out of people's mouths when cancer is sitting on the table. My hair falling out was the last thing on my mind. I was much more concerned with my impending demise.

Despite my wishes, word got around that I had cancer, and my face burned with shame. After all, what would people think? Now they would know how awful I was. I felt myself sinking into a slimy, black pit of despair. I stopped talking, eating, and sleeping— and pretty much everything else, too. *Why fight the cancer when cancer was exactly what I deserved?* I thought. I knew I was scaring my husband, Dan. I wanted to snap out of it, I really did, if only for his sake, but I couldn't. All I could hear was the voice inside my head that kept telling me I deserved to have breast cancer.

Wait a minute, this book is supposed to be about the *good* things, right? Although I didn't know it at the time, I was not in that pit alone. Another voice was speaking to me. I just couldn't hear it yet. Several years have passed since we first moved to Idaho, but I will always remember the day we arrived here. We came to Idaho because my husband, Dan, fresh out of graduate school, had been hired as a chemistry professor at Northwest Nazarene University, his first real job. He was thrilled, and I was plenty excited too, although it was harder to tell. My excitement was buried under a thick haze of exhaustion, the result of packing up and moving an entire household (including a cranky orange cat), as well as caring for a colicky newborn. Not only was I exhausted, but in this unfamiliar town, surrounded by strangers, I guess you could say I also felt pretty homesick.

That was before I met Lynn. If you took the wings off an angel, I am certain it would look just like Lynn. I could almost see the halo hovering above her head when she rang our doorbell that first evening in Idaho. In her hands she held a bucket of fried chicken, warm buttered biscuits, and chocolate chip cookies. I could have kissed her feet. She even brought paper plates and plastic forks in case our dishes and utensils had not yet been unpacked, which they hadn't. Holding our fussy little one, Lynn watched as I arranged the feast on a U-Haul box.

"We are so glad you and Dan and the baby are here," Lynn told me. "I served on the search committee that hired Dan. Every day since he accepted the position here at the university, I have prayed for you. And I am going to keep praying for you as you get settled into your home."

Saying exactly what I needed most to hear, Lynn, with her beautiful smile and her welcoming presence, filled our new home with grace that evening. All of a sudden I didn't feel quite so homesick anymore, and the task of unpacking did not seem as overwhelming. That night I rocked my baby till he fell asleep in my arms, all the while savoring Lynn's visit. These words of grace from a stranger were a gift of grace from God Himself.

Twelve years later, God called upon Lynn to once again deliver a gift of grace to me. Although the word was starting to get around, as far as I knew, Lynn had no idea I had been diagnosed with breast cancer. And, I had told no one about the "You-deserve-to-have-cancer" mantra on continuous re-play in my head. But God knew, and help was on the way.

Before I go on, perhaps I should make a small confession. The truth is that I have always found the Holy Spirit to be the tiniest bit annoying. I would be busy doing my own thing, checking items off my to-do list, and trying to accomplish more than I could realistically squeeze into one day. And then, the Holy Spirit would come and start nudging my heart. He would want me to call someone, make a meal, or do something else that I did not have time for, so I would try to talk Him out of it. Our conversations usually went something like this:

"Jill," the Holy Spirit would say to my heart, "The new family down the street needs you to make dinner for them tonight."

I would let out a huge sigh and roll my eyes. "But Lord," I'd whine. "I've got shirts to iron, letters to mail, and weeds to pull. And I'm a horrible cook! You know that I burn everything. Couldn't they just order pizza?"

Now, looking back, I realize it was silly to think that my to-do list was more important than God's. Lucky for me, Lynn was much better at following the Holy Spirit's guidance than I was.

I am not sure exactly how it happened, but I believe that the Holy Spirit asked Lynn to write a letter and told her exactly what to write. Amazing, right? But really, the part that amazes me the most is that Lynn obeyed Him and did it. I mean, if the Holy Spirit asked you to write a specific letter to a person regarding a rather personal and serious matter that you knew nothing about, would you be quick to get out the pen and paper? Not me! Oh, no, I would be sighing and rolling my eyes big-time. "Uh, how 'bout I just give her a call, Lord?" I'd say. "Or maybe I can ask around. Then if it seems like there really is a concern, maybe I'll think about writing that letter, okay?" Like I said, I am not exactly sure how it happened, but I do know that Lynn wrote that letter because she sent it to me.

I had already received a few "thinking-of-you" cards. But none of them had much writing on them because nobody really knows what to say to someone who has just been told she has cancer. So when a whole letter arrived in the mail from someone I didn't even know all that well, I was surprised and a bit curious. What did the letter say? I slit open the envelope and looked inside. Nothing could have prepared me for what I found.

Lynn's lovely handwriting flowed across the page. "Dear, dear Jill," she had written. "You certainly did not deserve to get cancer."

What in the world?! How could Lynn write that to me? I wondered. The voice in my head immediately clicked on and assured me that *yes, indeed, I most certainly did deserve to get cancer,* regardless of what was written in Lynn's letter.

As I continued to read, I noticed that Lynn had used the exact same words as the voice in my head, except she contradicted them. How could this be? Nobody else knew about that shameful voice.

That's when my arms got all goose-bumpy, and I realized that God must be speaking to me through Lynn. I felt like Moses may have felt when he figured out he was standing on holy ground. As I read Lynn's letter, God's glorious grace poured through me, His words washing away my feelings of awfulness and silencing, once and for all, that voice of condemnation in my head.

I read that letter over and over and over again. I kept it close to me for the next several weeks. After all, it's not every day that the mail brings a letter of grace straight from the heart of God.

In those first few days after my diagnosis, I remember a nurse asking me several questions to establish my medical history. One of the questions she asked me was, "Do you drink alcohol?" When I answered, "No," she looked up over her reading glasses and shook her pen at me. "Honey," she said, "if ever there is a time to start drinking, it's when you find out you have breast cancer."

That nurse was definitely right about one thing—I did need something to help me face this cancer ordeal. And God knew exactly what it was.

He knows what you need, too. Maybe there's no voice in your head telling you that you deserve to have cancer; but if you have been diagnosed with this disease, you are likely struggling with your own personal issues. God understands exactly what they are.
He wants to give you the gift of His grace, the wonderful grace we all need when our world turns upside down.

"For it is by grace you have been saved, through faith—and this is not from yourselves, it is the gift of God." (Eph. 2:8)

"Let us then approach the throne of grace with confidence, so that we may receive mercy and find grace to help us in our time of need." (Heb. 4:16)

"...My grace is sufficient for you, for my power is made perfect in weakness..."
(2 Cor. 12:9)

Practical Tip #1

God has sent a love letter to you, too. He has, in fact, sent lots of them. Take a break from reading those "How-to-Survive-Breast-Cancer" manuals and open your Bible. God knows what you need. Browse through Ephesians, Philippians, Colossians, and 1 John. These love letters are addressed to you.

2

COURAGE

Yea, Though I Walk through the Biopsy of Pain

It's no wonder that women dread their fortieth birthdays. Here we are, thinking about a triple-layered chocolate birthday cake surrounded by presents with fancy bows and happy people wearing party hats, when in reality on our fortieth birthday, we get smacked in the face with a big, honking mammogram. Fun? Not even close.

So there I was, on the examining table, wearing nothing but a gown made out of tissue paper. My doctor had completed my annual exam, and I must have passed because he said to me, "You know what, Jill? You are one of my healthiest patients. I know you're turning forty soon, but I think you could easily wait another year before you get your first mammogram."

Whoo-hoo! I wanted to jump up and shout with joy, but of course I didn't because of—well, you know—the paper gown thing. So I just said, "Really? Are you sure?" Then I got dressed as fast as I could and ran out of his office before he changed his mind, because he had given me the best birthday present yet. Or so I thought.

For the next few days, I celebrated my "no-mammogram-till-next-year" status— until my mother found out about it.

"It doesn't matter what that doctor said!" she informed me in that no-nonsense way that mothers have about them. "When you turn forty, you need to get a mammogram."

And so, reluctantly, I scheduled my very first mammogram because my mom told me to do so. I had no idea that she had just saved my life.

"It's no big deal, Jill," my mom assured me as I headed for the women's clinic. Funny, the mammogram technician said the same thing when I walked into the examining room: "It's no big deal."
But it was a big deal because, unlike a zillion other women who get mammograms each year, I had breast cancer. And that has to be the worst birthday present ever.

After evaluating my mammogram results, my doctor scheduled me for a stereotactic biopsy, which is really nothing more than a fancy name for "torture." Now to be honest, I talked to a few women (all breast cancer survivors) after I had this stereotactic thing; but instead of using words like "torture," they all described it with milder words such as "unpleasant" and "uncomfortable," which led me to the conclusion that I was an absolute wimp.

Of course, this was nothing new. As far back as I can remember, I have been a pitiful coward concerning medical matters. As a young girl, I often became sick with tonsillitis. My mom would take me to see the doctor, a soft-spoken man who attended our church. He wasn't so scary; but after he left the examining room, he always sent in a nurse to do his dirty work. Pretty sneaky, huh? The nurse would make me pull down my pants, and then she would poke my little bottom with an enormous needle, holding it firm until the thick penicillin meandered out. No amount of caterwauling on my part would speed up this dreadful process.

As a result of such painful medical practices over the years, I believe a whole generation of patients was created who, despite being sick, was too afraid to visit doctors. The medical profession has gotten much smarter now. Instead of using big needles filled with penicillin, doctors allow today's young patients to slurp down cotton-candy and bubble-gum flavored medicines; so I guess doctors will be staying in business after all. But it was too late for me. As far as I was concerned, the fewer doctors in my life, the better. Of course, that was about to change.

The stereotactic biopsy involves lying face-down and topless on a machine that was evidently designed to make the patient as uncomfortable as possible. The machine had no cushions, and the dips and curves were all in the wrong places. Because no adequate resting place was provided to accommodate my face, I was forced to twist my neck at an awkward angle. Oh, and did I mention that my breast was clamped in a vise and poked with sharp needles?

Perhaps the worst part of this procedure was the necessity to stay absolutely still, which was rather easy for the first two or three minutes. But each biopsy took an hour, and I had to have three of them. First, my foot started to itch; then my arms fell asleep. Before long, my neck developed the most awful crick. Unpleasant? This was way beyond unpleasant.

In order to stay as still as possible, I felt that I had to reduce my breathing to shallow breaths. However, a good forty minutes into the first biopsy, I started feeling light-headed, due, no doubt, to a lack of oxygen. I longed to gulp a mouthful of air and fill my lungs. Maybe I could take a slightly deeper breath without moving, so I decided to try. Ever so carefully, I gradually inhaled a teeniest bit deeper than I had been. Nobody would notice, right? Wrong, wrong, wrong. "Honey, if you do that again," said the radiologist, "we are going to have to start all over!" I decided that maybe I was getting enough oxygen after all.

Closing my eyes, I thought of my dear friend Ruthie, who had endured one of these biopsies herself a few years ago. She had shared with me how she had found comfort during the procedure by reciting the 23rd Psalm in her mind. That sounded like a good idea to me, so I began, "The Lord is my shepherd, I shall not want. He . . ." *Uh-oh, what comes next*, I wondered. Something about green pastures? Still waters? Come on, I have had this psalm memorized since I was seven years old! I racked my brain and finally came up with a line: "Yea, though I walk through the valley of the shadow of death." *Yes! That's me! I am in that valley right now, and death's shadow is looming over me!* But I could not remember another word of that beautiful psalm. I was stuck in the valley.

Three hours later, a technician escorted me to a different room. When I realized that she intended to give me a mammogram, I said, "You have got to be kidding. After three hours of mashing and poking my breast, now you are going to squeeze it in your mammogram machine?"

She wasn't kidding—not at all.

After completing the mammogram, the technician told me to sit in a chair while she took the pictures back to the radiologist. I sat there in that room, alone and completely topless, with blood seeping out of the multiple holes in my breast. The blood ran down my stomach, and I watched as it soaked into the waistband of my jeans. I remember thinking that I should grab some tissues to wipe up the blood and perhaps find one of those paper gowns to cover myself, but I could not move.

I was starting to comprehend what having breast cancer really meant. It involved much more than facing the possibility of my death. Having cancer meant walking through the valley of unpleasant and uncomfortable medical procedures. This biopsy only marked the beginning; many additional procedures loomed ahead of me.

I honestly did not think I could do it, not that I had any other options. If I gave up on the medical treatment, the cancer would spread throughout my body, and I would die a slow and painful death—not exactly an appealing alternative. I felt trapped in the valley, and nothing in my life had ever scared me more.

A while later, the technician returned to my room. As soon as she saw me, she set the papers she was carrying aside. Without saying a word, she took a blanket from the warming oven and wrapped it around my shoulders. Then she kneeled down in front of me and gently wiped away the blood and bandaged my breast.

While she silently cared for me, the rest of the words of the 23rd Psalm (KJV) at last came to my mind: "Yea, though I walk through the valley of the shadow of death, I will fear no evil: for thou art with me." Oh, yes, God was with me. I could feel His presence oozing over me like hot fudge on a sundae. Those words from the 23rd Psalm helped me realize that I did not have to endure those medical procedures alone. With God right there in the room with me, they did not seem quite so scary after all.

Breast cancer is not for wimps. God knows we can't run and hide. He understands that we don't have any other options. That is why He gives us the ability to confront the fear and the pain head on, all the while hanging onto the assurance that He is right there by our side. No matter how terrified we may feel on this journey, God is traveling through the valley with us. He gives us the gift of courage—the courage we need to walk right through the valley of the shadow of death.

" 'Have I not commanded you? Be strong and courageous. Do not be terrified; do not be discouraged, for the LORD your God will be with you wherever you go.' "(Josh. 1:9)

"For I am the LORD, your God, who takes hold of your right hand and says to you, Do not fear; I will help you." (Isa. 41:13)

"I will continue to rejoice, for I know that through your prayers and the help given by the Spirit of Jesus Christ, what has happened to me will turn out for my deliverance. I eagerly expect and hope that I will in no way be ashamed, but will have sufficient courage so that now as always Christ will be exalted in my body, whether by life or by death." (Phil. 1:18b-20)

Practical Tip #2
Even if you are confident in your ability to recite the 23rd Psalm, open your Bible and look it up. *Make sure* you have it memorized so that whenever you feel frightened in the days ahead, you can close your eyes, take a deep breath, and let the beautiful words of this psalm immerse you in comfort. Take courage in the assurance that God Himself is with you.

Practical Tip #3
If you have a low tolerance for torture and the nurse offers you a brain-and-pain-numbing pill before you undergo a procedure, don't hesitate to ask her for two.

3

HUMOR

A Time to Laugh

There is nothing funny about breast cancer. No matter how you look at it, breast cancer comes up one hundred percent non-funny every time. Scary? Yes. Painful? Yes. Funny? No. This is not a time to laugh but a time to cry.

During the first few weeks after my initial diagnosis, I underwent several medical tests and procedures to determine the extent and nature of my cancer. I quickly learned that if the test results were good, the nurse called me. If the results were bad, the doctor would call. During those first few weeks, the voice on the other end of my phone line always seemed to be my doctor.

The cancer was more extensive than originally thought, the doctor told me. We had not caught it early, and this was the invasive type. He talked about chemotherapy and radiation, and then he dropped the biggest bomb of all: a mastectomy.

Can you put a positive spin on a mastectomy? I didn't think so, but my doctor sure tried. He called it reconstruction and talked about it like it was a good thing, but I knew better. Reconstruction meant I would have to see yet another doctor and undergo more unpleasant and uncomfortable medical procedures.

Breast reconstruction is not a simple process. My doctor recommended that I see a plastic surgeon before my mastectomy surgery was performed to formulate a plan regarding the best reconstruction option for me. I had always thought God was the only one who could make something out of nothing. Apparently I was wrong since it seems that plastic surgeons can do so as well.

Now, I have nothing whatsoever against plastic surgeons; but if you would have told me a month earlier that I would soon find myself sitting in a plastic surgeon's office, filling out a form regarding nipple sensation and desired bra size, I would have said that you were absolutely crazy. Nevertheless, that is where I was and that's what I was doing. I could not possibly have been further out of my comfort zone.

My hands felt like ice as my husband, Dan, and I followed the nurse into the examining room. "A gown is hanging in the closet for you," she told me, "but don't put it on yet. The doctor would like to meet with you first."

A few minutes later, the doctor entered the room. He wore a suit jacket and tie and spoke in a distinguished, formal tone. I felt under-dressed for the occasion in my jeans and sweater. He introduced himself and carefully explained the various reconstruction techniques. While he spoke, he opened a drawer, took out a small white object, and laid it on the counter. Without making any reference to the mysterious white item, he instructed me to change into the gown and left the room.

I peeked in the closet, and was I ever impressed. No paper gowns here. Instead, I found a beautiful blue gown with gold buttons. Wow! Now, in the last few weeks, I had visited enough doctors to know the routine: strip off everything from the waist up. So that's what I did. When the doctor returned, I was wearing the lovely blue gown.

Maybe this won't be so bad after all, I thought.

The doctor took one look at me, put his hands on his hips, and scowled. "Well," he said, clearly irritated, "I guess you don't want to have reconstructive surgery after all!"

Did I miss something? I can't hear very well, so I looked to my husband for an interpretation of the doctor's strange behavior. But Dan was just as befuddled as I was. We stared back at the doctor like two nincompoops.

"Um, what do you mean?" I asked.

"This is what I mean!" the doctor sputtered, with both of his arms motioning to the white thing on the counter.

My husband and I are not ignorant people. Dan has a Ph.D, for goodness' sake! Yet we sat there, completely clueless. I stared at the white thing, hoping it might give me a hint. It looked like a surgical mask, the kind medical workers use to cover their mouths and noses. *Does the doctor want me to wear a mask?* I wondered. What is wrong with this guy? Doesn't he know that breast cancer is not contagious?

The doctor grabbed the white object and held it out for me to see. "If you want to have reconstruction surgery, then you have to wear this!" Then he put it back on the counter and left the room, shutting the door behind him.

Dan and I stood up and cautiously approached the white thing. I picked it up, and then it dawned on me. "I think I know what this is," I said. "It's a paper thong!"

Up until two seconds ago, I had no idea that paper thongs even existed. Dan watched in amazement as I tried it on. It was definitely not my style.

A while later, the doctor returned, not scowling this time; so I took that as a good sign. He told me to remove the blue gown, and stand in front of him wearing nothing but the thong.

"One way to reconstruct a breast is to form a mound on your chest wall by taking a section of fat from some other part of your body," he explained, all the while pinching, squeezing, and examining my exposed stomach, thighs, and buttocks in search of fat. Did I mention that I was way out of my comfort zone?

Then things got worse. When he finished pinching, he called his assistant into the room. She was carrying a camera—of all things. "We need 'before' pictures for your file," she explained. She set up a blue backdrop and instructed me to stand in various poses while she snapped away. I glanced at the crumpled gown lying on my chair and thought, *What is the point of having a fancy blue gown if they are never going to let me wear it?*

After what seemed like an extraordinarily long time, the assistant announced that we were finished. As soon as the doctor and the assistant left the room, I ripped off the paper thong and got dressed, grateful to be wearing my frumpy sweater and jeans again.

Dan and I exited the plastic surgeon's office in silence, perhaps because we were both in shock. Dan helped me into our car's passenger seat, then walked around the car, and climbed in on the driver's side. But he didn't start the engine. We both simply sat there, staring straight ahead. Finally, Dan turned to me and said, "Well, I guess one size fits all."

I turned to him, and our eyes met. And then I couldn't stop myself. Slowly I smiled, probably for the first time since I had found out about the cancer. Dan smiled back at me, and then we started laughing. We joked about the silly thong, the pictures, and the doctor's outrageous behavior until tears of laughter flowed down our faces. Laughter is a wonderful stress-reliever and anxiety-releaser. We needed that, but even more, we needed a new perspective on this cancer thing. We needed to find humor in the horror of the cancer journey.

There is nothing funny about breast cancer; yet in the midst of the turmoil inflicted by this wretched disease, God gives us the wonderful gift of laughter. He gives us a time to laugh because He knows we need it. And that is a good thing when you have cancer.

"There is a time for everything, and a season for every activity under heaven: A time to weep and a time to laugh." (Eccl. 3:1, 4a)

"She is clothed with strength and dignity [if nothing else!]; she can laugh at the days to come." (Prov. 31:25)

> *Practical Tip #4*
> **Whenever you're not sure whether to laugh or cry, always choose the laughter.**

4

FAITH

Got Faith?

When it comes to faith, I would have to say that the kids have it. How about adults? Bless our hearts, sometimes we don't even come close—not that it's our fault. You see, a little thing called reality often has a way of interfering with our faith. Kids don't seem to be affected by it the same way we are. Now, don't get me wrong; I am not saying that adults don't have remarkable faith. Over the years, the adults in my life have amazed me on numerous occasions with their incredible faith. It's just that sometimes reality sneaks up behind us and yanks our tail.

One thing I wish I could have known when I was first diagnosed with cancer was the devastating effect my bad news would have on those closest to me. Overwhelmed with concern for myself, I did not realize how heartbreaking my news would be to them.

Let's face it: telling family and friends that we have breast cancer is not easy. And to be honest, I expected them to react differently than they did. After all, I was too young for breast cancer, right? I figured they would deny such an absurdity, insisting that the cancer diagnosis was a mistake. I thought they might encourage me to get a second opinion or perhaps find a different doctor. I desperately needed them to wrap their arms around me and tell me everything would be okay, but nobody did. Reality says that breast cancer is a horrible disease, and despite our best efforts, it steals the lives of many, many women. I saw that reality reflected in the eyes of everyone close to me. I had a death sentence hanging over my head, and they were all horribly aware of it.

Perhaps I should have prepared them a little by telling them about the suspicious mammogram to give them all a heads-up that cancer might be coming for a visit. But at the time, my mom and I were planning a huge get-together for my dad's eightieth birthday. We did not have time for cancer; we were busy sending out invitations, sprucing up the house and yard, baking cakes, and blowing up balloons. It was a time for celebrating, laughing with friends, and catching up with family members we hadn't seen in a while. It was not a time to be worrying about the possibility of cancer.

Thus, it came as a powerful shock when a day or two after the party, my doctor called to inform me that I definitely had cancer. Forty minutes later, I found myself walking into my parents' house. My eyes were drawn to the rays of morning sunlight peeking in through their living room window. The soft light shone on my parents who were sitting in rocking chairs, both smiling and laughing as they looked at the photos we had taken at the party and reminiscing about the good time we had enjoyed. They looked up, pleased to see me. The scene was perfect, idyllic, and for a moment I considered not telling them about my cancer at all. The thought of speaking the word "cancer" out loud in the morning sunlight struck me as obscene and vulgar.

My mind often travels back to that moment as if it were suspended in time. Somehow I recognized it as my last moment of serenity before reaching the point of no return, leaving behind the comfort of life as I knew it and plunging into the frightening abyss of cancer. My voice sounded foreign to me as I spoke in my parents' quiet living room. "My doctor called this morning," I told them. "He says that I have breast cancer."

The words hung in the air, incomprehensible. My mom and dad continued to rock back and forth in their chairs, not saying a word or showing any emotion. Their silence continued for the next three days. Oh, sure, they made a few comments here and there regarding things like the weather, my kids' activities, and whether or not we should have pork chops for dinner. But for three solid days, not one word was said about my cancer.

In a way, their silence was oddly comforting. It led me to think that perhaps this cancer thing wasn't so bad after all. Their silence helped me endure those first difficult days.

When my parents finally did speak about my cancer, I realized how deeply upset they actually were. It occurred to me then that the only thing worse than finding out you have cancer would be finding out that your child does.

After that, I decided I had had enough of telling people about my cancer. Basically, I chickened out. I asked one family member and one close friend to share my news with those who were closest to me. However, three people still needed to be told about my cancer, and I knew I had to tell them myself. Those three people were my children. Of everyone, I dreaded telling them the most. Kaitlyn was seven years old at the time, Connor was nine, and Kyle was twelve. Not wanting to send them off to school feeling anxious and upset, I chose to tell them on a Friday afternoon. That way, we could spend the next few days at home together to discuss it.

"I have something bad to tell you," I said when they were all seated on the living room couch.

Kyle raised his hand. "On a scale of one to ten," he asked, "how bad is it?"

"This would be about a twenty," I told him. They all looked back at me with wide, worried eyes, and I felt myself choking up.

Connor broke the tension. "Come on, Mom," he said. "It's not like you have cancer."

Tears fell down my face as I nodded. "Yes, Connor, that is exactly what I have," I said. "Breast cancer."

I'm not sure what I had expected…perhaps an expression of shock or denial… maybe some crying or a hug…anything but a general lack of concern.

Connor looked doubtful. "How can you be so sick when you look just fine?" he questioned me.

Kyle nodded. "Yeah, you look perfectly healthy to me, Mom."

"It doesn't really matter anyway, Mommy," said Kaitlyn, standing up as if our meeting had been adjourned, "because God will make you all better."

And that pretty much settled the matter. This time I had overestimated the effect of my bad news. Cancer? Phooey. We had God on our side.

A week later, Dan took me to the hospital for my surgery. The doctor removed my breast, along with some other tissue and lymph nodes. That night in the hospital, I discovered the remarkable pain-reducing ability of morphine. After two days, my doctor approved my release, so I headed back home.

The forty-minute ride to my house turned out to be almost unbearable. My head spun, my stomach heaved, and my chest hurt. Kyle, Connor, Kaitlyn, and my parents stood waiting at home to welcome me when I finally arrived. No mirror was needed to tell me that I did not look good. I could barely stand, and the children watched as Dan helped me into bed. They saw my bandages and noticed my drains. They could see that I was in much worse shape than before I went into the hospital.

With my eyes closed, I could hear them whispering among themselves as they huddled around my bed, and I knew then that their faith was being tried. "Do you think Mom is really going to be okay?" they asked each other. "She looks pretty awful."

A day or two later, Kaitlyn walked into my bedroom and frowned as she looked me over. Although she did not say anything, her displeasure with the situation was obvious. Pretty soon, her lower lip started quivering. I thought I knew what would come next, so I reached out my hand to her. Boy, was I wrong.

Ignoring my outreached hand, Kaitlyn kicked my bed as hard as she could. Over and over again, she pounded the side of my mattress with her little foot. She was angry—angry at me for being so sick, and angry at God too, I think, for letting her down. Sobbing hard, she continued to kick. I could feel her doubt, discouragement, and fear with each jolt. Too weak to sit up, I simply lay there, with tears running down my face too.

I wanted to remind her of what she had so boldly spoken a week ago—that God was going to make me all better. But would He? I honestly did not know, so I didn't say a word. My little girl had to wrestle with this one on her own.

Kaitlyn's wonderful teacher, Mrs. Chandler, later shared with me a story she had written at school while trying to cope with the traumatic events occurring at home. Kaitlyn had called her story "Mighty Mom!" and this is what it said:

"My mom told me that she had cancer on a Friday, so I don't like Fridays anymore. She had her surgery on a Monday, and I

was really scared because Mondays usually don't go very well. But Daddy said the surgery went good, even though it was a Monday. I didn't see Mommy until Wednesday. She didn't look good at all. For six weeks she had to stay in bed. But then she got better and could get out of bed and back to doing her job of being a mom. I'm sure her next surgery will go good, but just to be safe, I hope it's on a Thursday, not a Monday, because Thursdays usually go much better."

A week or two after the bed-kicking episode, Kaitlyn marched back into my room. This time, she smiled at me. "Mommy," she said, sitting on the edge of my bed, "I've been thinking. God *is* going to make you all better, I'm sure of it. And when He does, we are going to have a big party to celebrate." She gently patted my hand, the matter of faith resolved.

There's nothing quite like the faith of a child, is there?

During this time of recovery, Connor did his share of writing too. He had learned about poetry from his teacher, Mrs. McConnel. She inspired him to write a "get-well" poem for me, a poem of faith. Connor called it "The Important Story," and this is what he wrote:

> *The important thing about Mom is she is going to get better.*
> *She is kind. She is pretty.*
> *But the important thing about Mom is she is going to get better.*

Connor read that poem to me at least six times a day while I recuperated. I think he wanted to make sure that I understood the part about getting better.

He also crafted an elaborate card on pink construction paper for me. The truth is, when I first saw the picture he had drawn on the cover, I was shocked. An unhappy stick figure labeled Dad was standing next to an equally unhappy but shorter stick figure labeled Connor, who was holding a bouquet of flowers. The most disturbing part of this drawing was the big headstone with the letters M-O-M written on it, as well as the stick figure with X's for eyes lying in front of this headstone. (**Note to self:** Do not encourage Connor to pursue a career in the "get-well" card business.)

A moment later, I noticed the big black X that Connor had scribbled over the whole picture, indicating an unacceptable scenario. Inside the card he had written, "Cancer is no big deal. Surgery is a part of life, not death. So now it is time to get well!"

My children insisted on believing that I would get better, despite my appearance to the contrary. Their faith refused to let them believe anything else. Each day they came into my room, checking for and expecting to see signs of my improvement. Nevertheless, those first few weeks after my mastectomy were tough for all of us.

One afternoon, my children gathered around my bed as I slept. Connor gently stroked my hand until I became aware of their nearness. Although groggy, I sensed their concern for me. "It's going to be okay," I whispered.

They shook their heads. "No," Kyle said. "You might die."

Possible death is the brutal reality of breast cancer, and it was staring me right in the face. How do you balance that reality with faith? I could think of only one way: by putting my faith in the One who had conquered death.

I looked at my children and their tears and said the hardest thing I have ever had to say to them. "Even if I die," I told them, "it is still going to be okay."

God's gift of faith surrounded us that day. More than ever, I felt sure of what we hoped for and certain of what we did not see.

Gradually, I did get better and stronger, eventually rising out of bed and getting back to being a mother again—just like my children believed I would. God gives each believer a measure of faith, but somehow it seems to me that the children get a bigger share.

I encourage you to accept God's gracious gift of faith, because whether or not we survive breast cancer, faith in God is the only thing that will ultimately save us.

"Now faith is being sure of what we hope for and certain of what we do not see." (Heb. 11:1)

"The only thing that counts is faith expressing itself through love." (Gal. 5:6b)

"Therefore we do not lose heart. Though outwardly we are wasting away, yet inwardly we are being renewed day by day. For our light and momentary troubles are achieving for us an eternal glory that far outweighs them all. So we fix our eyes not on what is seen, but on what is unseen. For what is seen is temporary, but what is unseen is eternal." (2 Cor. 4:16-18)

Practical Tip #5

Get yourself a faith box. It can be a fancy basket, a plastic storage bin, or a paper bag—whatever works for you. Fill your faith box with all the homemade cards, stories, pictures, and poems you receive. Look inside your box whenever you need to feel with your heart what you cannot see with your eyes.

5

HOPE

I Need a Hero

Ever since I can remember, I have had a big brother whose name is David. He is *not* a fireman. When I was five years old, my wonderful grandpa—a carpenter by trade—built a beautiful pink playhouse for me under the giant pepper tree in our back yard. Little girls from all around the neighborhood paraded down the sidewalk with their baby dolls to play in that house with me. Together we rocked our babies, changed their diapers, and fed them with those toy bottles that made it look like they were really drinking milk. We were in little-girl paradise.

But the fire changed everything. It started on the roof. First, we heard a crackling sound, then we saw the flames. As the playhouse filled with dark smoke, we grabbed our baby dolls and ran screaming out the door.

With a fireman's hat on his head, David rushed to the scene, gripping the garden hose. He bravely charged into the burning playhouse and doused that fire with water.

Because of his quick actions, my playhouse was saved. Oh, sure, a wall was charred, part of the roof needed to be replaced, and my plastic tea set had melted, but I had hope. My little-girl paradise could be restored, and it was all because of David.

From then on, I figured I could count on my big brother to rescue me, no matter what fires life brought my way. I grew up thinking of him as my hero.

Many years later, David and I, along with our spouses and children, gathered back at our parents' house for the Thanksgiving holiday. As we reminisced around the dinner table, I told the story of the playhouse rescue, starring my big brother.

But after all these years, the story sounded suspicious. Why was David already wearing his fire hat when the fire started? Was it a coincidence that he stood ready with the garden hose at the time of the fire? And how had the fire started in the first place? My hero had some explaining to do.

An expectant silence settled around the Thanksgiving table as we waited to finally hear the truth about the playhouse fire. David started with an apology. Then he explained how he had climbed the tree behind the playhouse and dropped shredded coloring book pages and burning matches onto the roof. I couldn't believe it: my hero was an arsonist.

It was probably just as well that I didn't know the truth back then because, as a child, it was good for me to have a hero in my life. Perhaps even adults need a hero from time to time. As I struggled to come to terms with my cancer diagnosis, I found myself wishing that my big brother could put on a fireman's hat and rescue me like he did when I was a little girl. I suppose, in a way, he did.

When I first found out I had a life-threatening illness, a mixture of thoughts flooded my mind, mostly concerns for my family. But an unexpected thought also taunted me: the realization that now I was going to die without ever having accomplished my dream of someday writing a book. I know that lots of people aspire to write a book, but for me it was my number-one dream, and my brother knew it. As a child, I had been crazy about writing, always creating a jumble of silly stories, poems, letters, and notes. As an adult, I have written hundreds of stories for magazines—but never a book.

Now, at forty years of age, I had cancer, and my dream was going up in flames. Yet my brother saw things differently. As we talked on the phone one evening, he said, "Hey, the good thing about all of this is that now you can write your book." It took a few moments for that to sink in. I mean, who says, "When I grow up, I want to get cancer so I can write a book about it"? Exactly no one, right? The more I thought about it, however, the more I realized that David could be right. I had always imagined that the book I intended to write would be fiction for kids, maybe teens. But hey, the subject of cancer might work in a non-fiction book for adults. Yeah, I could probably do that. In fact, I was now determined to do it.

Cancer changes everything. It shows no mercy as it stomps on treasured dreams, burns them up, and reduces them to ashes. But in spite of this, my brother reminded me that things could turn out okay after all. He had once again given me hope. Perhaps offering hope is what heroes do best.

Soon after my mastectomy, I returned to my doctor's office for a post-surgical exam. The exam was painful, and besides that, I still felt sick from the surgical anesthesia and drugs. But far worse than my physical distress was the emotional anguish I experienced because of the event that followed.

After the exam, Dan helped me dress. Then the nurse led us down the hall to a strange, little room and left us there. As I looked around, the first thing I noticed was the quiet—no phone, no clutter. Dust motes twirled in the filtered sunlight shining through the window. A simple book of flower poems lay on the table in front of me. Then I saw the box of tissues. That's when the purpose of this room dawned on me: this was the room of truth. At any moment, my doctor was going to walk into this room holding the preliminary pathology report from my surgery. The time of hoping for the best had come to an end. My future would soon be reduced to a few words of truth.

All of a sudden, I did not want to be there because I was not ready to give up hope yet. My heart pounded against my chest, and a sheen of perspiration broke out on my face. I needed air. Dan placed his hand on my arm, but I pushed it away. Feeling weak, I struggled to stand.

My attempt to run away was futile. Before I could take one step toward the door, the doctor entered the room. He smiled at me and spoke my name softly. I sat back down, feeling trapped and helpless. I just stared at the box of tissues.

The doctor sat across from me and opened my file. He went over the pathology report, using long and mysterious words that I didn't even try to understand. I figured that Dan could explain it all to me later. For now, I just kept my eyes focused on that box of tissues. When the doctor finally closed my file, I looked up. His eyes were fixed on mine, and I knew this was it—the moment of truth.

"Jill," he said in a gentle voice, "you have a rough year ahead of you, but when this year is over, I believe you will still be alive."

Alive? Really? I didn't realize I had been holding my breath until Dan squeezed my hand. I looked at him and saw that he had tears in his eyes. I probably did too. We were not going to need all those tissues after all because we still had hope.

The apostle Paul endured a lot of things during his lifetime, but as far as I know, he never had breast cancer. Even so, he sure knew a lot about pain, despair, and suffering. That much misery could cause anyone to become bitter and angry and want to give up hope, but not Paul. Over and over again, we read in the New Testament how he chose instead to put his hope in God. Paul knew the truth—that as long as we have heaven, we still have hope.

As I sat in that strange, little room soaking in the doctor's reassuring words, it occurred to me that even if he had given me the worst, most awful news, it could not have taken away my hope after all because years ago, I, too, had made the decision to put my hope in God.

Breast cancer is brutal. It relentlessly destroys dreams, desecrates families, and steals lives. If you have been diagnosed with this disease, then you know how impossible it is to stand up and confront the hopelessness of it all. We need help from a hero who will give us hope. Hope reminds us that it doesn't matter how bad things may appear from our point of view, because God knows how our story ends. And that is the very best we can hope for.

When we need a hero, God is always there for us.

"We wait in hope for the Lord; he is our help and our shield."
(Ps. 33:20)

"Remember your word to your servant, for you have given me hope. My comfort in my suffering is this: your promise preserves my life."
(Ps. 119:49-50)

"We rejoice in the hope of the glory of God. Not only so, but we also rejoice in our sufferings, because we know that suffering produces perseverance; perseverance, character; and character, hope. And hope does not disappoint us, because God has poured out his love into our hearts by the Holy Spirit whom he has given us."
(Rom. 5:2b-5)

> *Practical Tip #6:*
> You know that dream you've been hanging onto? Go pursue it!

6

PEACE

God's Powerful Peace

Located not far from my home is the Mountain States Tumor Institute. Most people around here call it MSTI, but to me it was "the-dreaded-place-where-people-with-cancer-have-to-go." I had never been inside the building or known anyone who had. Yet, for the past twelve years, every time I have driven past that place, chills have slithered up and down the back of my neck.

I always whispered a quick prayer for the cancer patients as I drove by. Then I would add a short but earnest prayer for myself: "Lord, for some reason, that place terrifies me. Please don't let me ever, ever have to go there."

Besides the obvious reasons, what scared me most about MSTI was that if I got cancer, I believed it would take away my peace—forever. It's not that I have ever been a particularly peaceful person. The truth is, I tend to worry about almost everything. So if I got cancer, I knew that it would take away the little bit of peace I did have. It would haunt me for the rest of my life because I would always be worrying about a recurrence. Any remotely suspicious pain, lump, or other symptom would send me scurrying back to the doctor. I would never be able to let it go and live my life in peace.

The day of my mastectomy dawned sunny and fresh, a beautiful spring morning that should have been enjoyed outside in the sunshine. I put on a brave front as Dan and I headed to the hospital, but I started getting nervous when we arrived at the parking garage. By the time we entered the hospital's huge lobby, my whole body was shaking. Why was I here? I felt perfectly healthy. Like an innocent prisoner, I was approaching the gallows. This was crazy. I should be running away from here, fast.

Then I noticed someone walking toward me. My friend Ann smiled and wrapped her arms around me. My anxiety faded away as she led Dan and me to a check-in area where her husband, Gary, stood waiting for us. Soon a few other friends joined us, as well as our pastor. It was starting to feel like a party, until a nurse came out and called my name. Dan and I moved toward her, but she put out her hand to stop Dan. "No husbands," she said.

My doctor had already explained that two hours before my surgery, I would undergo a procedure in which a radioactive dye would be injected into my breast--into the nipple, to be exact. He had promised me that Dan could be with me for this procedure and stay with me during the two-hour wait till my surgery.

One look at that nurse's face, and I knew I would have to resort to whining. "Please," I whimpered. "I really, really need my husband with me."

She didn't waver a bit. "Absolutely no husbands," she said. "Besides, it's only a little injection. We'll have you back here in a jiffy."

With that, she whisked me away from Dan, my friends, and the pastor without so much as a good-bye. The nurse led me along many corridors, through double-doors, and down stairways. Do hospitals have dungeons? That's where I imagined she was taking me. Eventually we came to a heavy door with one of those yellow and black signs posted on the outside warning about hazardous materials. Without hesitation, she ushered me through the door and instructed me to change into a hospital gown.

Soon the radiologist and a team of technicians entered the room. When they got out the needles, I understood the reason behind the strict "No husbands allowed" rule. If a husband had been allowed to witness that "little injection," he would have ended up passing out on the floor. I didn't fare much better.

After the procedure, I changed back into my clothes. Feeling shaky, I wanted to see Dan and feel his arms around me. I followed a nurse out into the hall, anxious to get back to the waiting room where Dan was.

Again, she led me through many corridors, and I lost all sense of direction. After a while, we passed through a set of double-doors and entered an area with a big sign that read "Pre-Surgery."

I grabbed the nurse's arm and stopped. "You were supposed to take me back to the waiting room."

She smiled sweetly, and I realized this was not the same nurse who had initially called me from the waiting room where I had last seen Dan. "What waiting room?" she asked.

"The one my husband is waiting in!" I cried.

She spoke to me as if I were a child. "This is a big hospital, and there are many waiting rooms. Let's get you ready for your surgery, and then I'll send someone to find your husband."

I never saw her again because she passed me off to a pre-op nurse, who took my arm and led me around a corner to a long hallway. Lining both sides of this hallway were many cubicles, each with a bed occupied by a patient awaiting surgery. The nurse stopped at the cubicle assigned to me.

"Here's where we'll get you ready for your surgery," she said.

I glanced inside my cubicle. The head of the bed had been shoved against the wall, and a muddle of medical equipment filled the rest of the space. It was so crowded that I could hardly find the floor. Thin partitions were all that separated me from the other patients. The nurse handed me a hospital gown. "I'll let you change into this," she said. "Then I'll be back to get you settled in the bed."

I watched as she whipped the curtain shut, giving me some privacy. Now, I am not a big person, yet I found it nearly impossible to change clothes in a space with barely enough room to stand. Also, I still felt shaky from my procedure. As I struggled to undress, I lost my footing, and my bare bottom fell past the curtain. Horrified, I yelped and scooted back inside my cubicle. Feeling my face start to burn, I hid behind the curtain. But there was no denying it: I had just mooned the patients across the hallway.

I quickly finished changing and might have crawled under the bed, but the nurse returned. She helped me up onto the bed and began preparing me for surgery.

"Have you found my husband yet?" I asked.

She looked puzzled. "Husband? I didn't see any men in the waiting room."

I tried to explain. "He's not in the pre-op waiting room. He's where I had my procedure."

"I'll see if I can find him for you," she said.

As soon as she finished prepping me, she left me all alone in that little cubicle in the middle of that big hospital, awaiting a surgery that would change my life.

After a while a young, good-looking guy, who looked like a technician of some kind, sauntered down the hallway. As he passed my cubicle, he turned his head toward me and gave me a goofy grin. I scowled back at him. Didn't he have any respect for a patient's privacy?

Soon he walked past and smiled at me again. *How annoying*, I thought. A little while later, he walked past yet again. What was his problem? Was he bored? Did they pay this guy a salary to annoy the patients? The fifth time he walked by, it occurred to me that maybe he had seen my bare bottom slip out from behind the curtain and now he was laughing at me. I wanted to scream. I mean, come on, I was just moments away from a traumatic breast surgery. What was wrong with these people?

My nurse returned. "Good news," she said. "Your doctor has arrived and is prepping for your surgery, and your operating room is all ready for you. It won't be long now."

"The only news I want to hear is that you have found my husband!" I snapped. I was feeling a bit cranky—can you tell?

She shrugged. "I'm sorry. We have been looking, but we still can't locate him."

"Then my surgery will have to wait," I informed her, "because I refuse to be operated on before I have seen my husband and prayed with my pastor!"

"I'll see what I can do," she said. "And by the way, your anesthesiologist will be here soon to go over a few things with you before your surgery."

She hurried away, and I was alone again. I stole a glance at the patients across the hall from me. They all looked so peaceful. What's the opposite of peace? No peace? That was exactly what I was feeling. Then that goofy, grinning guy came back down the hall again. But this time, he had the audacity to come right into my cubicle, hop up onto my bed, and reach for my hand.

"Hi, Jill," he said. "I'm Dr. Lavinski, but everyone calls me Dr. Love. I'm going to be your anesthesiologist."

I was speechless. Was this a joke? This was the guy who would be monitoring the oxygen flow to my brain? He would be holding my life in his hands while gawking at my bare chest during the operation?! Well! I certainly was not going to be calling him Dr. Love. I wrenched my hand out of his grip and reached over to yank the IV from my arm. I was getting out of here because I had definitely had enough of this place. I had no idea what that nurse had done with my clothes, but I would escape in my hospital gown if I had to.

My hand gripped the IV tube. As I started to pull, I heard voices and footsteps coming down the hall. The next instant, I saw my husband's face, and relief flooded through me. I let go of the IV tube, thinking that perhaps everything would be okay after all.

Dan and Pastor Johnson squeezed into my cubicle. Holding my hands, they prayed with me. A moment later, the OR crew arrived to take me away. The last thing I remember was hearing Pastor Johnson asking God to fill me with His peace.

A few weeks later, I found myself sitting exactly where for twelve years I had prayed that I would never be—in one of the examining rooms of "the-dreaded-place-where-people-with-cancer-have-to-go." As I sat in that cramped, windowless room waiting to meet my oncologist, I had nothing to do but stare at the IV equipment used to administer the chemotherapy drugs. I couldn't help thinking *why*. After twelve years of praying for God to spare me from cancer, why would He allow me to get it?

For nearly an hour, I waited in that small room, and as I sat there it slowly became clear to me. I knew that God had heard my prayers.

He cared about me, yet He had allowed me to get cancer anyway. God does not make mistakes, so my cancer did not take Him by surprise. He was in control, and I was in His hands. What better place could I possibly be?

How ironic that God would choose an examining room at MSTI to fill me with His peace. But doesn't that show just how powerful God's peace really is?

We don't have to let the threat of cancer haunt us for the rest of our lives; instead, we have another option. God wants us to live our lives in peace by placing our trust in Him. When we trust Him with our lives, He gives us the gift of peace. He sets us free from all the worries and fears that this hideous disease forces into our lives. God's incredible peace has the power to do that, and that is a good thing when you have cancer.

❧ ❧ ❧

"Now may the Lord of peace himself give you peace at all times and in every way." (2 Thess. 3:16)

"Peace I leave with you; my peace I give you. I do not give to you as the world gives. Do not let your hearts be troubled and do not be afraid." (John 14:27)

"From this time many of his disciples turned back and no longer followed him. 'You do not want to leave too, do you?' Jesus asked the Twelve. Simon Peter answered him, 'Lord, to whom shall we go? You have the words of eternal life.' " (John 6:66-68)

Practical Tip #7:
Time spent in the waiting room can be long and agonizing for your husband, friend, or parent. Before your surgery, consider asking a few members of your Sunday school class or perhaps your husband's close friend to stop by the waiting room for a brief visit. A small

care package of magazines and snacks might also be appreciated.

Practical Tip #8:

Become familiar with your treatment center. Many centers offer valuable resources such as access to a variety of breast cancer books and reference materials. Others offer affordable massages, exercise classes for patients undergoing treatment, and counseling services.

7

JOY

From Africa with Joy

Really, I should have been doing cartwheels, because I had just received the most awesome news yet: no intravenous chemotherapy and no radiation treatment! It was almost too good to be true.

In anticipation of the chemo, I had already cut off my long hair. In preparation for the radiation, my mom had purchased a few soft, button-up-the-front shirts for me, as well as some soothing cream to smear on my chest after the treatments. But now it looked as if I would need neither of those things.

Of course, my oncologist gave me a choice. I certainly could have chemo and radiation if I wanted them. After all, there was a chance that I would benefit from chemo. Also, even though my margins were clean enough not to necessarily warrant radiation, they were still very small. How do you make a decision like that? It was a tough call. A board of top oncologists reviewed my case. Their consensus was that in my particular situation, the harmful effects of chemo and radiation would likely outweigh the benefits. So they upheld my doctor's recommendation for no chemo and no radiation. I sure wasn't going to argue with that.

Like I said, I should have been doing cartwheels and celebrating my good news. The truth is that I felt immensely relieved and thankful, but was I happy? Not really.

Other people were happy for me. "Aren't you thrilled?" they would ask me while patting my back a little too hard. I would nod my head and mumble something about how perhaps the wonderful news needed a few days to sink in before it became real to me.

But after a week or two, I still did not feel anywhere near what anyone would call happy. As time went on, friends, family, and neighbors made comments such as "You never smile anymore" or "I haven't heard you laugh in a long time." They were right.

During this time, I experienced many sleepless nights. One night, since I wasn't sleeping anyway, I got up, grabbed a blanket, and curled up in the porch swing on our back patio. It was summertime, and since I have always enjoyed gardening, one of the ways I coped with my cancer was by planting tons of plants and flowers in the flower beds around our yard. I probably went a bit overboard; but hey, I had cancer, and if I needed to dig in the dirt and plant more flow-ers, no one was going to stop me. And truth be told, our yard did look pretty fantastic with all those flowers. In the daylight, it looked like an exploding rainbow. Yet as I sat out there in the middle of the night, a full moon gave the yard a cold, metallic look that filled it with dark shadows.

This is what my life has become, I thought to myself as the swing slowly moved back and forth, *void of color and warmth, void of happiness*. As I sat there in the dark, it occurred to me that cancer had taken away my joy.

For the next week, I concentrated on doing those things that had once brought me joy to see what would happen. I baked cookies for the neighbors, picked fresh flowers, visited with friends, listened to praise music, watched my favorite comedy movie, brushed the dog, ate chocolate, played the piano, and got a massage. Yet nothing worked.

I even tried spending extra time with three of my favorite people—my children. We played silly games and colored pictures with big, fat crayons. Together we read all our favorite children's books out loud, including *Morris the Moose Goes to School,* which we think is the funniest book ever. They burst into giggle fits and rolled on the ground, but not me. I felt nothing—absolutely nothing.

I didn't understand what was wrong with me because I had never suffered from depression or anything like this before. Remember the verse in Philippians that says to think about things that are true, noble, right, pure, lovely, admirable, excellent, and praiseworthy? It is one of my most favorite verses. I have always loved thinking about those kinds of things, but now my mind refused to cooperate. All I could come up with was a whopping, gray void.

In one last desperate attempt, I went to a restaurant and ordered a chocolate milkshake—the kind that comes in a fancy glass with whipped cream and sprinkles on top. I knew that I was in trouble after the first spoonful; I could just as well have been eating mud. My joy was gone, and I didn't have a clue about how to get it back.

Weeks later, I had a thought: I wondered if helping others could possibly bring joy to me. Dan and I support a thirteen-year-old girl in Africa through a Christian organization called Compassion. She and I have enjoyed writing letters back and forth ever since she learned how to write. I decided that I would send a special letter of encouragement to her, reminding her how much God loves her. After some careful thought, I chose to also tell her about my cancer.

I put the letter in the mail and did not think much more about it, till several weeks later when I received her reply. Can you put joy in an envelope and send it halfway around the world? That is exactly what this young African girl did.

Her letter oozed with love and concern for me, but that's not what brought me joy. What really touched my heart was that she had told *everyone* in her village about me, and all of them got down on their knees and prayed for me *every day*. Can you imagine? This rural African village, continually plagued by disease, hunger, and poverty, had been facing daily hardships that I cannot even begin to imagine, yet they got down on their knees in the dirt outside their huts every day to pray for *me*, a stranger who was concerned because she couldn't enjoy a chocolate milkshake anymore.

That young girl's letter went on to tell me how joyful and blessed her people were to be lifting me up in prayer. They believed that God would heal me, and they claimed that it was a joyous privilege to have a part in God's healing miracle.

That incredible letter reminded me that joy comes from the Lord—not from funny movies, fresh-picked flowers, or chocolate milkshakes. If all their tremendous hardships could not take the joy of the Lord away from those precious African people, then I surely was not going to let cancer take it away from me.

Looking to the Bible, which is jam-packed with verses about joy, I committed myself to spending time poring over its joy-filled passages. I refused to think about anything that made me feel unhappy and struggled to focus my mind on positive things. Daily, I asked God to help me by filling me with His joy. I sincerely believed that I would someday feel joy again; nevertheless, it was not an easy process, and it certainly didn't happen overnight.

During that time, I purchased a wooden plaque carved in the shape of the word "joy." It was probably meant as a Christmas decoration, but I kept it displayed on my desk where I could see it every day. It served as a reminder to me that, whether cancer likes it or not, joy comes from God.

Some time later, on a sunny autumn afternoon, I was riding in the back seat of my parents' car. We had been out running errands. As we got closer to home, I started gathering my packages together. I found a bag on the floor of the back seat that I didn't recognize and held it up.

"What's this, Mom?" I asked.

She turned her head to look. "Oh, that's the cream I bought for you to use after your radiation treatments." She smiled. "I'm glad you didn't need it after all."

I took the cream out of the bag and read the label. I could not believe it. "You bought me *Udderly Smooth Udder Cream*?" I asked her. "Mm-hmm, it's a great moisturizer."

She didn't get it. "Mom," I said, starting to laugh, "do you realize you picked *udder* cream to moisturize *my* udders!"

Come on now, that's funny, isn't it? I passed the bottle of cream up front so she and my dad could read the label for themselves. I could not stop giggling.

As my parents and I laughed together in the sunshine, I felt the warmth and color gushing back into my life. I'm a bit sketchy on the mechanics of it all, but I strongly suspect that the Holy Spirit was involved.

I was able to smile and laugh again. I definitely felt something, and I was pretty sure it was joy.

That evening, my children and I went for a walk. Watching the vibrant, changing colors of the sunset, I realized I had received yet another gift from God—a gift that came through a beautiful young girl on the other side of the world who shared with me the joy of the Lord.

≈   ≈   ≈

"Our mouths were filled with laughter, our tongues with songs of joy. Then it was said among the nations, 'The LORD has done great things for them.' The LORD has done great things for us, and we are filled with joy." (Ps. 126:2-3)

"You have made known to me the path of life; you will fill me with joy in your presence." (Acts 2:28)

"He will yet fill your mouth with laughter and your lips with shouts of joy." (Job 8:21)

"The joy of the Lord is your strength." (Neh. 8:10b)

> ### *Practical Tip #9:*
> Borrow or buy a pretty robe and soft button-up shirts to wear during treatments. Treat yourself to a manicure or pedicure. Dab on some of that perfume you've been saving for a special occasion.
>
> ### *Practical Tip #10:*
> Be kind to yourself. Think positive, gentle, and loving thoughts.

8

PERSEVERANCE

Keeping Your Chin Up

My dad was never one to show much sympathy. I remember a night when I called home from college during my freshman year. My boyfriend had just dumped me like yesterday's trash, and although it was one of the best things that ever happened to me, at the time I felt devastated. I called home in hopes of telling my mom the sad story, but she wasn't there. My dad informed me that she would not return home till later. Disappointed, I did the next best thing. I spilled out the whole story to my dad. And do you know what he said when I finished? "Keep your chin up." That was it. No soft, soothing words of comfort—or anything.

That's what he always said when life got tough. As I was growing up, he never once let me feel sorry for myself.

During my three pregnancies, I experienced awful morning sickness. I threw up everywhere I went—in the grocery store, at the park, in my doctor's office, and even once in the neighbor's flower bed. While I was pregnant with Kaitlyn, our youngest, the church secretary asked me to bring dinner to a visiting missionary couple. Boy, was that ever a mistake. Too sick to cook, I ordered pizza. Dan and our two little boys came with me to help deliver the food, and the kind missionary couple insisted that we all join them for dinner. As we gathered around their dining room table and helped ourselves to the pizza, I kept thinking, *This is not a good idea.* Sure enough, without any warning whatsoever, I threw up all over their dinner table and the pizza. No one at church ever again asked me to bring dinner to any missionaries.

Many people sympathized with me and tried to help me through the morning sickness problem, but not my dad. More than a few times, he would smile and pat me on the shoulder like he was congratulating me or something. "Jill," he'd say, "this morning sickness is a great opportunity for you to learn perseverance!"

And that's a *good* thing? I found it impossible to share his enthusiasm. All through my pregnancies, he kept encouraging me to keep my chin up. Only after I got breast cancer did I realize that perhaps perseverance was a good thing after all.

Lab test results indicated that my cancer was estrogen-receptor-positive, so my oncologist recommended hormone therapy. He prescribed tamoxifen, an innocent-looking pill that I would swallow every day for the next five years. An older breast cancer survivor from my church assured me that taking tamoxifen was just like taking a vitamin. Oh yeah? Well, no one warned me that for a *pre*-menopausal woman whose ovaries were still spewing out ginormous gobs of estrogen, taking tamoxifen can be just like having your body twisted inside out and left hanging upside down.

My voice shook when I called my oncologist. "Something is wrong!" I told him.

"Tamoxifen has many possible side effects," he calmly assured me. He read me a long list of them. "Which side effect are you experiencing?"

"ALL of them!" I shouted.

Hot flashes, fatigue, bone pain, joint aches, constipation *and* diarrhea (yeah, I didn't think that was possible either), headaches, insomnia, indigestion, lack of appetite, irregular menstrual periods, and mood swings were the side effects I was experiencing. But the worst by far was the nausea. Even the *thought* of food could start me retching. Entering a grocery store, sitting in a restaurant, seeing a food commercial on TV, or even hearing someone say the word "food" made me sick.

Since the rest of my family still wanted to eat three meals a day, this presented quite a challenge. Even if someone else did the cooking, I could not tolerate the smell of food in the house. At first people tried to help by bringing us meals, which we greatly appreciated, but we needed to find a solution that would have to last for perhaps the next five years.

My husband tried to explain this all to my oncologist at my next check-up appointment. "Ever since Jill started taking tamoxifen, it's like I'm married to someone who's pregnant and taking a crash-course in menopause at the same time."

The oncologist responded by prescribing more pills to help me cope with the side effects; however, each pill had its own list of side effects which, in many cases, only added to my misery.

Cancer-survivor friends recommended certain vitamins and health foods, but it took months to determine which of those would work best for me. I read books and articles and scanned the Web, trying to learn as much as I could about how to cope with tamoxifen's nasty side effects. But it still was not easy; it took perseverance.

During this miserable time, my dad sent a special e-mail to me. I was surprised to receive his e-mail because, for one thing, my dad hardly ever sent long personal e-mails to me. Also, he hardly *ever* talked about the time when he, a young South Dakotan farm kid, was drafted into the Army to fight in the Korean War. I read his e-mail shortly after dawn while the rest of my family slept.

Dearest Jill Diane,

This is your dad. It is early morning. I could not sleep any longer, so here I am. After I woke up and had my personal devotions, my thoughts were of you. These thoughts brought to mind an old memory of 54 years ago, my first day in Korea.

We, my comrades and I, had had a long day. Early in the morning we had disembarked from the landing ship in the Inchon harbor of Korea and boarded an unheated train car. The first part of the journey was through the rubble that had not too long ago been Seoul, then on through the damaged and scarred countryside. It was winter, so the day was short. When darkness fell, we boarded open 6x6 trucks. Around midnight we arrived at the rendezvous area from which our 40th Division would take over from the 24th Division. Big squad tents had been set up: no heat, but some protection from the wind and cold night air. Former rice paddies, frozen and badly-rutted, served as our floor. Here, we experienced our first introduction to the roar of the artillery shelling in the distance.

But a better part was that there was mail waiting for us, mail that had arrived while we had been en route from Japan. Many did not receive a letter, but there was one for me. It was from my dad, your grandpa—a very short note in his good handwriting. A few flashlights were passed around so we could read our mail inside our sleeping bags to hide the light. Your grandpa had few pleasantries, considering the stress and anxieties of the situation. His closure meant the most to me. He told me, "Keep your chin up."

And now I say the same to you, dear Jill. Keep your chin up.

Much love to you,
Dad

Never before had I considered what a miserable and frightening experience it must have been for my dad and those other teenage boys to be taken away from their rural farming town and shipped overseas to fight a war they probably did not much understand. For forty years my dad had been encouraging me to keep my chin up.

Now I finally understood why that phrase meant so much to him. After eight months of struggling with the side effects of tamoxifen, I received the shocking news that my healthy, strong dad had been diagnosed with cancer. He had a rare form of lung cancer called mesothelioma, which is caused by exposure to asbestos some twenty, thirty, or even forty years earlier in life.

His prognosis was not good. For the next seven months, he fought the cancer, endured the pain, and persevered without complaint. But this was not a fight he was going to win.

I stayed with him during his final week of life. One afternoon as I sat quietly next to his bed, he caught hold of my hand. "How am I doing?" he asked me with a weak smile. I knew he was dying, but I could not bring myself to say the words. So I smiled back, squeezed his hand, and whispered, "You just keep your chin up, Dad."

Four days later, he died.

Life improved somewhat for me after that first rough year on tamoxifen. In some ways, I think my body adjusted to the drug. Or perhaps, the pain of losing my father made the physical maladies seem less significant.

But I realize now that I never would have made it through that first year if I had not learned how to persevere, a gift God gave me years ago through my wonderful dad.

"Blessed is the man who perseveres under trial, because when he has stood the test, he will receive the crown of life that God has promised to those who love him." (James 1:12)

"As you know, we consider blessed those who have persevered. You have heard of Job's perseverance and have seen what the Lord finally brought about. The Lord is full of compassion and mercy." (James 5:11)

"You need to persevere so that when you have done the will of God, you will receive what he has promised." (Heb. 10:36)

Practical Tip #11:

You will likely develop relationships with others who have cancer, and they may not all survive. Write it on the back of your hand if you have to, or post a banner across your bathroom mirror, but do whatever it takes to remind yourself as often as necessary that it is okay to be the one who survives.

Practical Tip #12:

Remember that you are stronger and more resilient than you may think.

9

PATIENCE

Feeling a Bit "Discomboobulated"

It happened in the Albertsons supermarket down the street from my house. As I reached down to grab a can of black olives off the bottom shelf, my heavy gel prosthesis slipped out of my bra and out of the top of my shirt and plopped unceremoniously onto the floor of the condiment aisle.

Now, I have received a lot of advice during my lifetime, but nobody has ever told me what to do when your prosthesis splats like a piece of raw chicken onto the floor of Albertsons. For a moment, I considered leaving it there and kind of nonchalantly walking away. But then I imagined some gallant stranger picking it up and saying, "Hey, lady, you dropped your, uh . . ." How embarrassing would *that* be? So instead, I snatched it up and shoved it into my purse. Without making eye contact with any of the other shoppers, I ditched the can of olives and made a swift exit.

That settled it—no more putting it off. The olive incident served as my notification that the time had come for me to start the reconstruction process. This meant that I had to go back to see the plastic surgeon, back to the place with the little paper thong.

An appointment was scheduled, and a few weeks later I found my-self sitting in the plastic surgeon's examination room. This time, much to my delight, I actually got to *wear* the lovely blue gown. The plastic surgeon, in his suit and tie, stood before me, pontifi-cating about the various reconstruction techniques. After much discussion, Dan and I decided that an implant would be the best option for me. This procedure would require three surgeries. First, an expander would be surgically placed under the skin where my breast used to be. That surgery would be followed by a series of weekly visits to the plastic surgeon's office for "fills," in which a needle would be used to inject a small amount of saline solution into the expander. When my skin had stretched and expanded enough to provide room for the implant, the surgeon would perform my second surgery. In this surgery he would remove the expander and replace it with the implant. The third and final surgery would involve a skin graft to form the nipple.

Sounds simple enough, right? It was, except that I felt ready for my new breast much sooner—as in immediately. But that was just not to be. My surgeon pointed out that I would need a good three or four months to heal between each surgery. He estimated that the reconstruction process would take close to a year. I tried to sigh quietly.
As our meeting came to a close, the plastic surgeon stepped for-ward and shook my hand. "Ms. Nogales," he said, "you are going to get your new breast, but it is going to take time. You are going to have to be patient."

Then he turned me over to his three medical assistants who looked just like—I'm not kidding—a set of modern-day Charlie's Angels. At first I felt intimidated by these perfectly beautiful women, but they smiled kindly at me. "It's going to be okay, Jill," one of them assured me. "We are going to be your new best friends."

They were right. The four of us spent a considerable amount of time hanging out together as we inspected various sample implants and tried to determine what type, shape, and size would be the best match for me. It was almost like shopping for just the right pair of shoes, but not quite.

Once these decisions were made, I was eager to proceed. (Well, I was eager to get it over with, actually.) My first reconstructive surgery was scheduled for as soon as possible which, unfortunately for me, was a full two and a half months away. This, of course, meant that I would have to be patient.

When the day of my surgery finally arrived, I showed up at the hospital feeling a bit apprehensive. Because the needles, queasiness, and pain of my previous operation still remained fresh in my mind and since I am not particularly fond of such things, I felt nervous about undergoing another surgery. A nurse prepped me for the operation and then let Dan chew his fingernails with me till the time arrived for me to go to the operating room.

While we waited, my plastic surgeon popped into my cubicle. I honestly did not recognize him. Gone were the formal tie, the crisp white shirt, and the dark jacket. Instead, he wore loose-fitting scrubs and a poofy hair-net thing. On his feet were big surgical fluffies. I almost expected to see little bunnies on them.

Even his eyes were smiling as he greeted me with exuberance. "Hi, Jill! Good to see you!"

He approached me with a magic marker, of all things. The nurse helped me stand and remove my hospital gown. Then the surgeon took that blue marker and doodled all over my chest, drawing dotted lines, circles, and arrows. All the while, he chatted about what an exciting day this was. I stood there, amazed. His enthusiasm and optimistic attitude were contagious, and I felt myself relaxing and laughing with him. This man in the scrubs was in his element, doing what he did best. Now I understood why he was so highly recommended.

The surgery went well. After a few weeks of recovery, I was back on my feet and making my weekly visits to Charlie's Angels for fills. We quickly determined that my skin was very thin and delicate, so it was not strong enough to handle a normal fill. The doctor/plastic surgeon tried injecting only half the amount of saline solution. That seemed to work, but it meant that the lengthy filling process would take twice as long. I tried to be patient.

At last the doctor determined that my skin had sufficiently stretched, so we scheduled the next surgery. Now we were getting somewhere. Dan and I showed up at the hospital, the doctor did his thing with the magic marker, and then he performed the surgery that switched the expander with my new implant. Pretty exciting, right? I had to wait a few weeks before the bandages were taken off and the swelling went down so I could actually see my new breast, but it was worth the wait. I finally saw a glimmer of light at the end of the long, dark cancer tunnel, or so I thought.

It soon became apparent that my skin was just not strong enough to hold the implant in place, which was slowly slipping down toward my waist. Disappointing? Yes, but my doctor assured me that we would do another surgery to try to fix it. The trouble was that we would have to wait at least two more months to allow my body to finish healing. Did I mention that I was trying to be patient?

Then, something happened three days later that would require even more time for my body to heal and much more patience. It was mid-morning on a weekday when I headed out to run a few errands. I was on a major road with six lanes, three in each direction with a divider separating them. I drove in the center lane of the traffic flowing in my direction. Although the light ahead of me was green, the traffic in my lane was stopped. Yet, traffic in the lanes on either side of me clipped along at a good thirty to forty miles per hour.

Then, I saw him in my rear-view mirror. He was jabbering on his cell phone as he roared up behind me in a shiny, white three-quarter ton pick-up truck. I thought that perhaps he had his eye on a break in the traffic, so I expected him to swerve into the lane to either the right or left of me. But he didn't. Instead, with no sign of any attempt to slow down, he crashed into the back of my old mini-van, smashing the entire front end of his truck. The impact threw me forward, slamming my chest against the steering wheel and knocking the wind out of me.

A police officer appeared seemingly out of thin air right there at the scene of the accident. He and the driver of the white truck, who was apparently unhurt, rushed to help me out of the van. As they opened my door, a gush of chaos surrounded me—cars, people, noise, and exhaust. Yet I was aware of only one thing: I could not breathe.

Grabbing my cell phone, I pushed the quick-dial button to call my husband's office. When Dan picked up, I could hear his voice on the other end of the line, but I had no breath with which to speak to him and no way to tell him I needed his help.

The officer walked me to the curb and helped me sit down. He kept asking me, "Are you hurt? Shall I call the paramedics?" I could not give him an answer because I was still struggling to breathe.

Desperate to fill my lungs, I fought to gulp in as much air as I could. As my breath slowly returned, I became horribly aware of one other thing; I was indeed hurt. The impact of the collision had definitely injured me. Clutching my chest in pain, I realized that the accident had wrecked my reconstructed breast.

Did I need this? Hadn't I already suffered enough? First, I had breast cancer and a mastectomy, then reconstruction and tamoxifen, and now I've been hit by a *truck*? Really? Just because some careless guy had been talking on his cell phone when he should have been paying attention to his driving, my reconstructed breast was now destroyed?!

I felt as if little explosives were detonating behind my eyeballs. Surely

I had reached the point where my brain was categorizing this latest event into the "THAT'S TOO MUCH!" category. Huge sobs burst from deep inside me, and tears flooded my face. I paced back and forth on the sidewalk while leaning forward, holding my chest, and wailing in agony. I was out of control, hysterical, and distraught. It was not my finest moment.

I almost felt sorry for the truck driver and the police officer. They both seemed bewildered by my behavior and apparently had no idea what to do with me. They followed me awkwardly as I walked back and forth, afraid to touch me or leave me. The officer kept insisting that I should be examined by a paramedic, but I adamantly shook my head. The last thing I needed was yet another man looking at my scarred and battered chest.

I probably should have explained to them about the breast cancer and my recent mastectomy, and that I was still recovering from reconstructive surgery; and now I was very upset because this crash had messed it all up. Yet, I did not want to discuss my private parts with these strange men because it was none of their business. So, I stubbornly refused to tell them anything.

Not knowing what else to do, the policeman called in a female officer. When she arrived, she helped me call my husband and tell him what had happened.

"I'm coming right now," Dan said. "Where are you?"

For the first time, I looked around at my surroundings. St. Luke's Hospital, where I had undergone my first two reconstruction surgeries, stood right before me. "St. Luke's," I told Dan.

This was a big mistake. Dan thought I was actually *in* St. Luke's as a badly injured patient in the emergency room, barely clinging to life. No wonder he arrived at the scene of the accident so quickly. He looked somewhat relieved when he found me standing in one piece on the street in front of the hospital. I guess that in comparison, the actual trauma of my situation seemed rather minor to him in light of what he had been imagining on his drive to St. Luke's.

I was calming down and starting to accept my current state of affairs. The female police officer still wanted to involve the paramedics, but I explained to her that they were not going to be able to help me because I needed the expertise of my plastic surgeon.

Have I ever told you that my husband is a brilliant man? He pointed out that since the crash had taken place very close to my plastic surgeon's office, we should go there right away. Undoubtedly, the male officer and the truck driver blew out a huge sigh of relief as Dan helped me into his vehicle and drove me away.

The medical staff at the office greeted me with great care and concern, and the surgeon graciously agreed to see me at once. Dan helped me change into the blue gown, and then the surgeon gently examined me. My reconstruction was definitely in bad shape: the implant had been ripped completely loose and was now free-floating under my skin. Gravity insisted on pulling it down to my waist. Was it painful? Incredibly so, and quite unattractive by any standards. I wanted it fixed immediately, yet my surgeon did not agree. He assured me that I would be okay; but before he could do anything to fix the problem, my chest required lots of time to heal—not only from the most recent surgery, but now from the accident as well. I had no other choice but to wait it out.

I became well acquainted with painkillers. Time passed slowly, but the plastic surgeon was right. I finally did get my new breast. I'm not saying that he did a better job than God, but the end result was well worth waiting for.

Patience has never been one of my strengths; I am so much better at complaining. But consider this: our God is a patient God. So if we desire to become more like Him, it follows that we also need to develop patience, right? Of course, no one ever said that would be easy, but I believe it's possible with the help of the Holy Spirit.

Perhaps the best way to develop patience is when we have no other choice, and that is a good thing when you have cancer. Welcome or not, it provides an opportunity for us to learn how to be more patient, one day at a time.

ع ع ع

"Be joyful in hope, patient in affliction, faithful in prayer."
(Rom. 12:12)

"But the fruit of the Spirit is love, joy, peace, patience, kindness, goodness, faithfulness, gentleness and self-control. Against such things there is no law." (Gal. 5:22)

"Therefore, as God's chosen people, holy and dearly loved, clothe yourselves with compassion, kindness, humility, gentleness and patience." (Col. 3:12)

Practical Tip #13:
Sports bras, worn even while you sleep at night, offer comfort and support as your body heals during the reconstruction process.

Practical Tip #14:
Appreciate each day. Life may not always be good, but it's certainly better than the alternative.

10

FRIENDSHIP

A Little Help from Our Friends

Have you noticed yet that most of the people around you have a problem spitting out the word "cancer"? It's like saying the word "bomb" on an airplane. Folks just aren't comfortable with that. Instead, they use hushed voices to murmur phrases like "serious illness," "health issues," or "medicinal treatments" as if the word "cancer" is an obscenity that's too hideous and offensive to speak out loud.

But cancer is what it is. Giving cancer an "it-which-must-not-be-named" status only adds to its fearfulness and contributes to a pitiful attempt of denial. Yet, that's what many people do—even friends.

Not all of my friendships survived my cancer experience. When they heard about my diagnosis, a few friends shrunk away from me as if I had contracted some foul, pus-oozing infection. I haven't heard from them since, which may be just as well. Not everyone can handle the unpleasantness of cancer.

Then there were the friends who couldn't get enough of my cancer. Every day they would call to get an update on my condition, appearing to savor the grisly details. To them, my life was a soap opera, and they were eager to pick up the phone and tune in to the next shocking episode. I got the feeling that some were disappointed to hear that I wasn't already in a coffin.

But thankfully, plenty of friendships have remained that were strong enough to withstand the cancer; in fact, they have become stronger despite the cancer. These friends are no less than precious gifts from God Himself, and I consider their relationships among the good things I encountered as I stumbled along my cancer journey. Three years before I was diagnosed with breast cancer, Dan and I decided that our growing family needed more room to—well, grow. We chose to build, so we purchased a lot, hired a draftsman to draw up house plans, and contracted with a builder.

We visited the construction site almost daily, eagerly watching as our new home took shape. I often looked around our soon-to-be new neighborhood, and I grew curious about the people living inside the houses. Were they friendly? Would we have anything in common? Would we become friends?

I never had a sister. Perhaps we would have fought, argued, and pulled each other's hair; but nonetheless, I felt it was my loss not to have had one. As I looked around the new neighborhood, I realized that it must be full of women. Maybe I could develop a close relationship with one of them—not as a sister, of course, but more like as a special friend. She might be one who lived close enough that we could borrow a cup of sugar from each other or spend a lazy summer afternoon sipping lemonade on the back porch. I got excited about the possible opportunities, so I began praying. For the next few months as our house was being built, I asked God to provide a special woman friend for me in the new neighborhood. I didn't care if she was young or old, a stay-at-home mom or a career woman. I believed that God would answer my prayer and trusted that He would find just the right person for me.

Soon after we moved into our new house, a neighbor brought us a plate of home-made sugar cookies. I wondered if perhaps she was going to be my new friend. Another neighbor offered to watch our children while we carried in some heavy furniture, and I couldn't help wondering if maybe she was going to be my new friend.

After six months of playing this "Are-you-my-new-friend?" game with my neighbors, it seemed the answer was a big, fat no. It's not that I wasn't making friends and developing relationships with the new neighbors. It's just that none of them felt like the special friendship for which I had prayed.

During this time, Terri Slemmer, one of my best friends, had put her house up for sale. With six children, she and her husband Duane were also looking for room to grow. They were considering several larger houses, one of which was a few houses down the street from ours. My family and I were thrilled when they decided to buy the house in our neighborhood. Our children were good friends, our husbands both worked at Northwest Nazarene University, and we attended the same church. This was going to be great fun, being neighbors and all.

Okay, you might be thinking this is pretty obvious, but I just didn't get it at first. For the next few months, I continued looking for my "new" friend. Eventually it dawned on me that *Terri* was the answer to my prayer. Instead of making one of the neighbors become my new friend, God had arranged for one of my friends to become my new neighbor. Awesome, huh?

I thanked God for the wonderful answer to my prayer. I greatly enjoyed the special relationship I had with Terri and her family, but I had no idea just how important this friendship was to me till I found out I had breast cancer.

It still amazes me that God knew all along how my family and I were going to need the Slemmers in the worst way. Two and a half years before I even knew I had cancer, he put them in place to minister to me and my family.

From the moment that I found out I had a suspicious mammogram, Terri was in this cancer thing right along with me. In fact, her entire family was our number-one support group. They reached out to us in many important ways, and because they were our neighbors, they were able to minister to us much more effectively than if they had lived farther away. To tell you the truth, I'm not even sure of all the many things the Slemmers did for us. But I do know they were always there when we needed them, and they helped us through the awful cancer experience in countless, and often thankless, ways.

They were not the only ones. Our friends Kamela and Dan Lawrence were also there for us every miserable step of the way. They kept us well supplied with food, flowers, and hugs.

It was a tradition for the Lawrences and my family to watch the Super Bowl game together at our house. However, when the Super Bowl fell on a day less than a week after one of my reconstructive surgeries, I figured that we would have to break that tradition. But the Lawrences were not going to let us do that. First, they suggested that we come to their house to watch the game; but I wasn't strong enough, and I was too selfish to let Dan and the kids go without me. So then, they decided to bring the party to us. Kamela, who can fix the most awesome food, brought a truckload of it to our house and assumed the role of hostess during the entire game. My Dan kept me on schedule with pain pills so that I felt good enough to join most of the party, even though I may have drifted off to sleep once or twice in the recliner. I sincerely hope I didn't drool, but even that would have been okay because the Lawrences graciously accepted this situation as if it were not the slightest bit awkward. Only really good friends can do that, and the Lawrences are some of the best.

Then there was Nikki Pearsall. Nikki's lovely mother had been diagnosed with breast cancer some years ago, so Nikki was familiar with the whole cancer scene. She knew what we needed and when we needed it, and she always gave it with a sunshiny smile. I am convinced that Nikki has a direct link with the Holy Spirit, divine ESP, or something like that because she was incredible. I remember one evening when I felt overwhelmed with fatigue and nausea. I knew that Dan would be home from work soon and the kids were already getting hungry, but I felt too sick and weak to make supper for them. So I did the only thing I could do: I prayed. "I need help, God," I whispered. "Please provide dinner for my family." And the very next second, that's right, *the very next second*, the doorbell rang. There stood Nikki, smiling and holding a delicious, hot meal for us. She did this over and over and over again. I would put in a desperate call to God for help, and the next second Nikki would appear at my front door holding the answer.

Some long-distance friends also touched my life and ministered to me in amazing ways. Mary Beth Roossien, who had been one of my best friends ever since the days we shook rattles together and crawled around the church nursery in our diapers, refused to let the fact that we lived on opposite sides of the continent stop her from helping me. She sent cards, flowers, and care packages. Even though I had not seen her in years, her words of encouragement touched me deeply and helped me heal.

Another long-distance friend, Amy Nichols, also ministered to me in a remarkable way. Amy and I had met during our freshman year of college. A special friendship developed between us, and we ended up being roommates for the next three years. We kept in touch throughout the years since college, and when she found out I had cancer, she wanted to do something special for me. She planned a "girls" weekend for just the two of us. While our husbands watched the kids, she flew to Idaho, rented a plush hotel room, and asked me to meet her there. For two whole days she pampered me. We ate the finest chocolate, went to a day spa for pedicures, and dined at one of those fancy fondue restaurants. It was wonderful.

But perhaps the best thing she did for me was listening. That's right;

she sat there in the hotel room with me and listened as I spewed out all the bad things about cancer. Once I got started, I could not stop, and it was kind of scary because I held nothing back. The words flowed from my mouth like a raging river. For two days I vented all the horrible, awful things cancer had caused me to suffer. It's a wonder that her ears didn't shrivel and fall off her head!

I guess I had thought I could make this whole cancer experience a little less traumatic for my children, family, and friends if I bottled up the bad stuff by smiling and saying, "I'm fine!" Not very smart, huh? I was not very good at it, either. I'm sure I didn't fool anyone, and certainly not Amy. That "girls" weekend was the best thing she could have ever done for me because it allowed me to let go of the bad stuff.

Hanging out with me as I dealt with cancer could not possibly have been much fun for my friends. During that time, I'm sure that I was not much of a friend to any of them. Even though I wanted to be, I was in survival mode, so that's all I could handle. Yet they stuck by my side, holding my hand through the most difficult times, giving me comfort and strength, and helping me heal. That's what true friends do.

Friends like the Slemmers, the Lawrences, Nikki, Mary Beth, and Amy, as well as the many others who ministered to me and my family with their friendship, don't just happen. They are gifts from a loving heavenly Father who anticipates and understands our needs better than we ever could.

Filled with the Holy Spirit and guided by God's Word, friends are able to touch our lives and meet our needs in inconceivable ways. I believe that God equips our friends, who are created in His image, to tangibly bring His tender loving care right to our doorsteps and into our hearts when we need it the most. Let's face it: when we have cancer, we could all use a little help from our friends. That is a good thing.

❧   ❧   ❧

"For he will command his angels concerning you to guard you in all your ways." (Ps. 91:11)

"Do not forsake your friend and the friend of your father, and do not go to your brother's house when disaster strikes you—better a neighbor nearby than a brother far away." (Prov. 27:10)

"If one falls down, his friend can help him up." (Eccl. 4:10)

Practical Tip #15:
Take pictures (or ask someone to take them for you) of the flowers, gifts, and even the food you receive. These visual aids will be helpful later as you write "thank you" notes.

Practical Tip #16:
Now may be a good time to consider resolving any negative relationships in your life.

11

COMPASSION

The Gift That Keeps on Giving

In the beginning, I never had a shortage of people to talk with regarding my cancer. My husband, my mom, a few close friends, nurses, and doctors all listened attentively as I tried to process and accept my cancer diagnosis. They were immensely helpful, but it wasn't enough for me. Something was lacking because none of them had ever actually had breast cancer. I felt a great need to talk to someone else—someone who had experienced breast cancer first hand and lived to tell about it.

A mutual friend put me in touch with a woman named Jan who had gotten breast cancer twice and survived. This incredible woman called me at home, and for forty-five minutes she openly shared her cancer experience with me and answered all my intrusive questions. I felt grateful for all the information and advice she gave me. But before she hung up the phone, she added one more comment that I found rather disturbing. I had thanked her for sharing her story with me, and she replied by saying, "Jill, now it's your turn to share your story with others and encourage them as they go through their cancer experience."

Was she crazy? I had just found out about my own cancer! I had no idea how or if I would survive this myself, so I could not possibly imagine ever helping someone else.

Soon after my phone conversation with Jan (the very next day, in fact), women started flocking to me. They would tell me about a worrisome lump in their breast and ask if they should get it checked. Others would tell me about a suspicious mammogram and ask if I thought they might have cancer.

Because I had no clue about what to say to them or what they wanted from me, I longed to cover my ears and run away. I could hardly be considered an expert, since my *only* experience with a suspicious mammogram was that it definitely meant cancer. Is that what they wanted to hear? Their stories terrified me because I figured they must all have cancer too, just like I did, and we were all going to die. I mentioned this to my mom. "Why are all these women telling me about their breast problems?" I asked her, hiding my face in my hands. "Some of them have never even talked with me before. What do they want from me?"

Although my question consisted of mostly rhetorical whining, my wise mother provided an answer. "Well, you could listen to them," she said. "You could pray for them and share their concern."

I nodded. Yeah, I could probably do those things, but I didn't really want to. I didn't believe I had anything to offer.

Two years later, I sat at my desk and wrote out a check. After sealing it in an envelope, I marched out front and put it in the mailbox. It was my last cancer payment. Even with good insurance, I had discovered that cancer is pretty stinking expensive. For the past two years, all the money that should have been paying for fun family trips to Disneyland, new tires for the van, and other important things like food went instead to pay off the hospitals and my numerous doctors, including the radiologist, the pathologist, the anesthesiologist, and more.

But now the last payment had been made, and I felt free. I was finally going to put this nasty cancer experience behind me and forget it ever happened. In fact, we were not ever going to mention the "C" word again.

The next day, the phone rang. A friend from church was calling me in tears. She had just found out that she had breast cancer. To be honest, my first instinct was to slam down the phone. I did not want to revisit that painful time in my life by reliving that first horrible day when the doctor had told me I had cancer. Yet, I could tell that she was scared and upset. She had questions and hoped I could provide some answers. For the first time, I realized that maybe I could. Determined to help my friend, I went back in my mind and thought about what I had needed most that first day. More than anything, I had needed someone to tell me that everything was going to be okay—that even though cancer is an awful, horrible disease, my family and I would make it through this experience. That's all I had needed to hear, even if it wasn't the truth.

So that is what I told her, in a way, but I mainly listened. I reassured her that even though cancer was bad, she was going to be okay. We stayed in close contact over the next several months, and I had the privilege of walking with her through her valley. I would like to think that I somehow made the experience a little less awful for her, but I can't take credit for that. I believe God did that by giving her gifts like grace, courage, and peace along the way, just like He did for me.

Remember Jan, the cancer survivor who had encouraged me to share my story two years earlier? Well, I finally realized she was right. At the time, I hadn't recognized her wise words for what they were, but now God had given me one more gift: compassion. I now had compassion for women everywhere who have been shocked by those horrible four words, "You have breast cancer."

Sharing my story has not been easy. In fact, writing it down has brought forth more tears than the actual experience did. But sharing is good. Stories make us strong because they encourage us and give us hope. They remind us that we are not alone.

Perhaps someday you will be ready to share your own story. When that time comes, I hope that God will give you the gift of compassion. I believe your compassion can bring strength and encouragement to other women whose worlds have been turned upside down. That is a good thing that can come out of cancer.

"I will tell of the kindnesses of the LORD, the deeds for which he is to be praised, according to all the LORD has done for us—yes, the many good things he has done for the house of Israel, according to his compassion and many kindnesses." (Isa. 63:7)

"Therefore, as God's chosen people, holy and dearly loved, clothe yourselves with compassion." (Col. 3:12a)

"All of you, live in harmony with one another; be sympathetic, love as brothers, be compassionate and humble." (1 Pet. 3:8)

> ***Practical Tip #17:***
> Consider keeping a journal to record your thoughts, prayers, and meaningful Bible verses. Or, if you prefer, express yourself through art or music.

12

LOVE

As High as the Heavens

A few weeks before cancer invaded my life, in the quiet of the afternoon before my children got home from school, I knelt beside my bed and prayed. This was no trite, rattled-off prayer but a serious, down-on-my-knees, Hannah-like prayer. I had a special request to make known before God.

Even now, I am not at all sure why I made that particular request. As far as I can remember, no problem, concern, or fear prompted it. Looking back, I wonder if I would have had the courage to make such an earnest request had I known how God was going to answer it. The day that my doctor called to tell me I had cancer also happened to be the same day that Dan and I had been planning to celebrate our eighteenth wedding anniversary. Arrangements had been made in advance for the kids to sleep over at my parents' place, and Dan and I had special plans to enjoy a fancy dinner and romantic night together—just the two of us.

However, our much-anticipated evening did not turn out as I had hoped. Cancer tends to have that effect on even the best of plans. My parents still picked up the kids, who, unaware of my bad news, were excited about the slumber party with Grandpa and Grandma.

When Dan came home from work, he brought a dozen red roses for me. In shock, he and I spent the evening staring at the roses, hanging on to each other, and wondering how, after eighteen years of marriage, our lives had come to this.

The first time Dan and I ever saw each other was at the beginning of our freshman year of college when I rode past the men's dorm in my roommate's red Ferrari. He says it was love at first sight. (I'm still not completely sure if he was referring to me or the car!) Nevertheless, a year later, he asked me out on our first date. We dated throughout our sophomore year and continued to see each other during our junior and senior years. Our college was located in beautiful San Diego, and when we weren't studying, Dan and I took long walks along the beach, explored the city, had picnics in the park, and watched the sunset over the ocean. Those were some of the happiest years of my life.

We got married a year after graduation. I followed Dan to Reno where he had been accepted into the doctoral program at the University of Nevada, Reno. Graduate school can be brutally tough on marriages. During our five years there, we watched the marriages of more than a few of our grad school friends crumble into divorce. But our marriage survived and grew stronger, despite the stress and pressure of those years.

Soon after Dan finished graduate school, our first baby was born. Three years later, we had another. Two years after that we had our third. While I nursed babies and changed diapers, Dan worked hard to develop his career as a chemistry professor and a researcher. Those were busy, demanding, and often downright hectic years. I have heard that some marriages drift apart or explode during such times, but not ours. Dan and I stayed close to each other. Perhaps that's how it works when you marry your best friend.

And now, looking back, I guess you could say we had pretty much made it. Our three kids were all in school and doing well. Dan had established an enjoyable and fulfilling career at Northwest Nazarene University, and I was busy writing. We had a great home and a great marriage. Life was good.

So I honestly have no explanation for why I got down on my knees that one quiet afternoon and asked God to bring Dan and me even closer together. Maybe I just wanted more of a good thing. Perhaps I believed, with God's blessing, that our marriage could become even greater. Whatever the reason, I asked God to bump our love for each other up to the next level.

Although I had no doubt that God would answer my prayer, I never imagined His answer would come with a diagnosis of breast cancer. Don't get me wrong, I am not saying that God caused my cancer, but I do believe He allowed my prayer to be answered through the cancer.

There is nothing like a terminal disease to bring relationships and values into sharper focus. Some issues that may have been really important to us suddenly become insignificant in light of a cancer diagnosis. On the flip side, other things that we may not have paid much attention to or have taken for granted become of the utmost importance.

I had always thought that Dan and I would grow old together, but now I wasn't so sure. "Till-death-do-us-part" means when we're really old and wrinkled, right? It's surely not when we reach forty! Dan and I were life partners. How could death possibly consider separating us, right in the middle of our lives?

As I tried to come to terms with the fact that I had cancer, I scoured the Bible, searching for any verses that might provide comfort and understanding. Psalm 103 became my favorite passage. Of course, I loved the part in verse 3 that says God "heals all your diseases." But my favorite part by far was verse eleven, which says, "As high as the heavens are above the earth, so great is God's love for us."

When my children were younger, I used to read them a children's bedtime book called *Guess How Much I Love You*, by Sam McBratney. This wonderful story illustrates the immeasurable love that exists between a parent and a child. As the story unfolds, no matter how much Little Nutbrown Hare says he loves the Big Nutbrown Hare, it seems that the Big Nutbrown Hare always loves him more. At the end of the book, the sleepy Little Nutbrown Hare says, "I love you right up to the moon." The Big Nutbrown Hare agrees that that is very far. Then he lies down next to the little one and whispers, "I love you right up to the moon—and back."

Verse 11 in Psalm 103 reminded me of that book. Whenever I read that verse, it was like God was telling me, "This is how much I love you, Jill, all the way to the heavens— and back." I figured if God loved me that much, I could make it through anything, even cancer. God made His love real and tangible to me through my husband, Dan. Soon after my diagnosis, Dan surprised me by purchasing an expensive bottle of perfume for me. Cashmere Mist by Donna Karan was my most favorite cologne, not that I had ever actually owned some of it. It wasn't *that* expensive, but I had just never made it a habit to indulge in department store perfumes before this. But when Dan found out I had cancer, he bought a big bottle of Cashmere Mist for me.

Dan had, of course, bought many gifts for me over the years, but this one was extra special. Cancer had made me feel worthless, tainted, and ugly. But Dan's gift of expensive perfume made me feel that even if I was dying, I still had worth and value; and most important of all, it made me feel loved.

I dabbed on some Cashmere Mist every day, even on the days when I was only going to the store or cleaning the house. The scent served as a constant reminder that even if cancer could separate us, it could never take away Dan's love for me.

One afternoon, Dan and I were driving home from one of my doctor's appointments. We were almost to our house when Dan stopped the car because standing in the middle of the busy road was a male Mallard duck. Other cars were beeping their horns, but the duck didn't seem to notice. All his attention was focused on an object lying in the middle of the road. As we looked closer, we saw that it was a female duck. Apparently, she had been hit by a car. She had not survived. Yet, her devoted partner stayed with her, trying to comprehend the terrible loss that had occurred. We slowly drove around the duck. When we ran an errand an hour or two later, the male duck was still there—still standing in the middle of that road, still oblivious to the honking cars, and still watching over the lifeless body of his mate.

They were ducks, I know that. Yet Dan and I could not help wondering if cancer could do that to us.

If there is one thing I have learned from having cancer, it is that you are not in control. You may like to think you're in control; but when you get cancer, the one thing that is crystal-clear is the fact that you are not, and never have been, in control.

So when I got cancer, Dan chose to do the one thing that he could do: he chose to love me. Do you know what that kind of love looks like? It empties your surgical drains. It stays awake all night watching over you, and then still goes to work the next day. It never complains. It goes to every doctor visit, every exam, every procedure, and every surgery. It waits patiently during recovery. It does not dwell on how its own needs are not being met. It holds hands, it hugs, and it whispers words of love. It never gives up hope.

When things were at their worst, Dan made a promise to me. He promised me that when this was all over, he would take me to Hawaii. At the time, I'm not sure I believed him, or maybe I thought I would be making the trip in an urn. But Dan kept insisting that I was going to get better, and that when I did, we would make the trip together. His loving promise encouraged me and helped me through even the darkest days.

Two years later, I found myself lying in the sunshine on a beautiful beach in Maui. Dan had fulfilled his promise. Together we celebrated our twentieth wedding anniversary there in Hawaii, just like he had promised me.

At the beginning of this book, I mentioned that the extraordinary gifts God lavishes on us—grace, peace, courage, and more—are the good things that can happen when we have cancer. But the very best gift that God gives us has got to be the gift of His love. Of all the gifts that I have talked about in this book, I believe this one is by far the most important. God loves you. That's nothing new, right? But when you get cancer, God pulls out all the stops, and I mean *all* the stops. He lets His love pour over you in astonishing and unfathomable ways. His love flows to you through those around you. It may flow through your husband. Maybe it will flow through someone else close to you —your mom or dad, a sister or friend, your pastor, a co-worker, a nurse, or a neighbor. No matter who it flows through, reach out your arms and embrace that love. It is yours for the taking as a gift from our wonderful God. His love never fails. His love knows no limit. It reaches as high as the heavens. And that is a good thing when you have cancer.

"And now these three remain: faith, hope and love. But the greatest of these is love." (1 Cor. 13:13)

"I pray that you, being rooted and established in love, may have power, together with all the saints, to grasp how wide and long and high and deep is the love of Christ, and to know this love that surpasses knowledge—that you may be filled to the measure of all the fullness of God." (Eph. 3:17b-19)

"How great is the love the Father has lavished on us, that we should be called children of God! And that is what we are!" (1 John 3:1a)

> ### *Practical Tip #18:*
> The one-year anniversary of your mastectomy, lumpectomy, or end-of-treatment is a significant milestone. Plan a party to celebrate life. Invite your friends, family, neighbors, pastor, doctors, and nurses to celebrate with you. Thank them for being a special part of your life.

Jill Nogales

Jill Nogales

CPSIA information can be obtained at www.ICGtesting.com
Printed in the USA
267391BV00002B/1/P